HIGH

FIBER

FOOD LIST

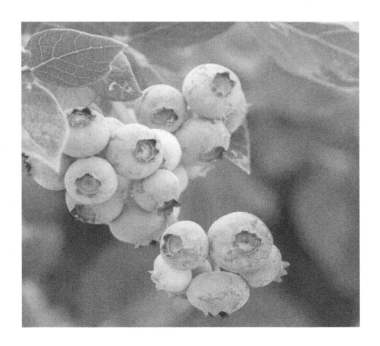

LORENE PEACHEY

DISCLAIMER

The content within this book reflects my thoughts, experiences, and beliefs. It is meant for informational and entertainment purposes. While I have taken great care to provide accurate information, I cannot guarantee the absolute correctness or applicability of the content to every individual or situation. Please consult with relevant professionals for advice specific to your needs.

TO GAIN ACCESS TO MORE BOOK BY THE AUTHOR SCAN THE QR CODE

TABLE OF CONTENTS

INTRODUCTION..1

CHAPTER 1 7

What is Fiber?..7

   Importance of High-Fiber Foods: 8

CHAPTER 2 11

Recommended Daily Fiber Intake..11

   General Guidelines for Recommended Daily Fiber Intake: 11

   Age and Gender-specific Recommendations:.......................... 12

CHAPTER 3 15

High-Fiber Vegetables 15

CHAPTER 4 21

High-Fiber Fruits...21

CHAPTER 5 25

Whole Grains...25

CHAPTER 6 31

Legumes and Beans...31

CHAPTER 7 37

Nuts and Seeds...37

CHAPTER 8 .... **43**

Fiber-rich Snacks **43**

CONCLUSION **49**

BONUS CHAPTER 1 .... **51**

10 HIGH FIBER RECIPES **51**

BONUS CHAPTER 2 .... **68**

21 DAY MEAL PLAN **69**

INTRODUCTION

In the vibrant tapestry of life, my journey as a nutritionist has been a kaleidoscope of flavors, a symphony of nutrients, and an exploration of the profound impact that food choices can have on our well-being. Hello, dear reader! I am Lorene Peachey, your guide through the gastronomic realm of health and vitality. For the past 25 years, I have dedicated my life to unraveling the secrets of nutrition, and today, I stand before you as an advocate for the transformative power of high-fiber foods.

Imagine a world where each meal is not just a source of sustenance but a celebration of life, where every bite fuels your body, nurtures your spirit, and paints your soul with the vibrant hues of well-being. This is the world I've been exploring, a world where nutrition becomes an art form, and dietary choices are the brushstrokes that create a masterpiece of vitality.

My fascination with nutrition began as a quest for answers to simple yet profound questions. What if the food we eat could not only satiate our hunger but also elevate our mood, boost our energy, and fortify our resilience against the challenges of life? What if our plates held the key to a healthier, happier existence? These questions stirred my curiosity and ignited a passion within me to explore the alchemy of food.

Picture this: a kitchen filled with the aromas of fresh herbs, the sizzle of vibrant vegetables in a pan, and the promise of a meal that not only tantalizes the taste buds but also nurtures the body. This is where my culinary journey began—where I transformed the mundane act of cooking into a delightful symphony of flavors and nutrients, weaving together the science of nutrition with the artistry of culinary creation.

As I delved into the world of dietary research, one crucial element emerged as a hero in the nutritional narrative—fiber. This unassuming, often overlooked component became the protagonist in my quest for a healthier lifestyle. High-fiber foods are not just ingredients; they are the unsung heroes of our well-being, providing benefits that extend far beyond the plate.

Now, let me pose a question that might awaken a sense of curiosity within you: Have you ever considered the impact of your daily food choices on your overall health? Our lives are a series of choices, and what we put on our plates is no exception. In a world where convenience often trumps nutrition, where fast food beckons with its tantalizing flavors, we find ourselves at a crossroads. The choices we make today can either lead us down the path of vibrant health or into the labyrinth of lifestyle-related ailments.

Consider this: what if I told you that incorporating high-fiber foods into your diet could be the transformative key to unlocking a healthier, more energized version of yourself? The benefits of a high-fiber diet are like a treasure trove waiting to be discovered. Imagine having more energy, improved digestion, and a reduced risk of chronic diseases—all within reach, just by embracing the rich tapestry of high-fiber foods.

Let's dive into the core of this nutritional treasure chest. Fiber, the unsung hero, comes in two forms—soluble and insoluble—each playing a unique role in promoting our well-being. Soluble fiber, found in foods like oats, beans, and fruits, helps lower cholesterol levels and stabilizes blood sugar. On the other hand, insoluble fiber, present in whole grains, nuts, and vegetables, adds bulk to our stool, aiding digestion and preventing constipation.

But the benefits of high-fiber foods extend beyond the digestive system. Imagine waking up each morning with a sense of vitality coursing through your veins, knowing that the fiber-rich choices on your plate are supporting your heart health. High-fiber foods have been linked to a reduced risk of cardiovascular diseases, acting as a shield against the number one cause of mortality worldwide.

Now, let's delve into the emotional realm. Have you ever experienced the exhilarating feeling of sustained energy throughout the day, free from the energy crashes that often accompany processed, low-fiber meals? Picture yourself effortlessly navigating the demands of your daily routine, fueled by the long-lasting energy that high-fiber foods provide. Imagine the joy of indulging in a meal that not only satisfies your taste buds but also supports your mental and emotional well-being.

The emotional benefits of a high-fiber diet are profound. Studies have shown that consuming fiber-rich foods can positively impact mood and reduce the risk of depression. As we nourish our bodies, we nourish our minds, creating a harmonious balance that transcends the boundaries of physical health.

Now, let's discuss the dark side of the culinary universe—the consequences of a diet dominated by processed, low-fiber foods. Picture the chaos within your body as it struggles to process the onslaught of refined sugars, unhealthy fats, and empty calories. A diet lacking in fiber can lead to weight gain, sluggish digestion, and an increased risk of chronic diseases. It's a slippery slope into a realm where convenience trumps nutrition, and the toll on our health becomes increasingly evident.

Consider the following questions: How does your body feel after indulging in a meal high in processed foods? Do you experience a surge of sustained energy, or is it followed by a wave of fatigue? How about your digestive system? Does it operate smoothly, or do you often find yourself grappling with bloating and discomfort?

Now, imagine a different scenario—a scenario where your meals are not just a means of survival but a source of vitality. A high-fiber diet can be your compass in navigating this culinary landscape, guiding you toward choices that not only taste good but also make you feel good from the inside out.

As I stand before you with 25 years of experience in the world of nutrition, I invite you to join me on a gastronomic adventure where high-fiber foods take center stage. My journey, marked by countless experiments in the kitchen and a relentless pursuit of nutritional wisdom, has culminated in a curated list of high-fiber recipes that transcend the mundane and elevate the act of eating to an art form.

Picture yourself savoring a quinoa salad with chickpeas, a symphony of textures and flavors that nourish your body and delight your taste buds. Envision the comfort of a lentil soup, each spoonful a testament to the power of whole foods in promoting health and vitality. Imagine the satisfaction of biting into a sweet potato and black bean taco, a culinary creation that not only satiates your appetite but also fuels your body with the nutrients it craves.

As we embark on this journey together, my mission is clear—to empower you with the knowledge and tools to make choices that resonate with your body's needs. The high-fiber food list I present to you is not just a compilation of ingredients; it is a manifesto for a life well-lived, a celebration of the incredible machine that is your body.

Contact the Author

Thank you for reading my book! I would love to hear from you, whether you have feedback, questions, or just want to share your thoughts. Your feedback means a lot to me and helps me improve as a writer.

Please don't hesitate to reach out to me through

lorenepeachey@gmail.com

I look forward to connecting with my readers and appreciate your support in this literary journey. Your thoughts and comments are valuable to me.

CHAPTER 1

WHAT IS FIBER?

Fiber, also known as dietary fiber or roughage, is a type of carbohydrate found in plant-based foods that the human body cannot digest or absorb. Unlike other carbohydrates, such as sugars and starches, fiber passes through the digestive system relatively intact. There are two main types of dietary fiber: soluble and insoluble.

1. **Soluble Fiber:** This type of fiber dissolves in water and forms a gel-like substance. It can help lower blood cholesterol levels and regulate blood sugar levels. Good sources of soluble fiber include oats, barley, beans, lentils, fruits (especially apples and citrus fruits), and vegetables.

2. **Insoluble Fiber:** This type of fiber does not dissolve in water and adds bulk to the stool. It aids in preventing constipation and promoting regular bowel movements. Whole grains, wheat bran, nuts, seeds, and the skins of fruits and vegetables are rich in insoluble fiber.

Importance of High-Fiber Foods:

1. **Digestive Health:** High-fiber foods promote a healthy digestive system by preventing constipation and promoting regular bowel movements. Insoluble fiber adds bulk to the stool, making it easier to pass through the digestive tract.

2. **Weight Management:** Foods high in fiber tend to be more filling, which can help control appetite and prevent overeating. Additionally, high-fiber diets often have lower calorie density, contributing to weight management.

3. **Heart Health:** Soluble fiber helps lower blood cholesterol levels by binding to cholesterol molecules and removing them from the body. This can contribute to a reduced risk of heart disease.

4. **Blood Sugar Control:** Soluble fiber can help regulate blood sugar levels by slowing down the absorption of sugar. This is particularly beneficial for individuals with diabetes or those at risk of developing diabetes.

5. **Colon Health:** High-fiber diets are associated with a lower risk of developing colorectal cancer. The bulk provided by fiber helps move waste through the colon more efficiently, reducing the time harmful substances are in contact with the colon lining.

6. **Prevention of Chronic Diseases:** A diet rich in fiber has been linked to a lower risk of various chronic diseases, including type 2 diabetes, certain cancers, and cardiovascular diseases.

7. **Improved Gut Microbiota:** Fiber serves as a prebiotic, nourishing beneficial bacteria in the gut. A healthy balance of gut microbiota is associated with better overall health, including a strengthened immune system.

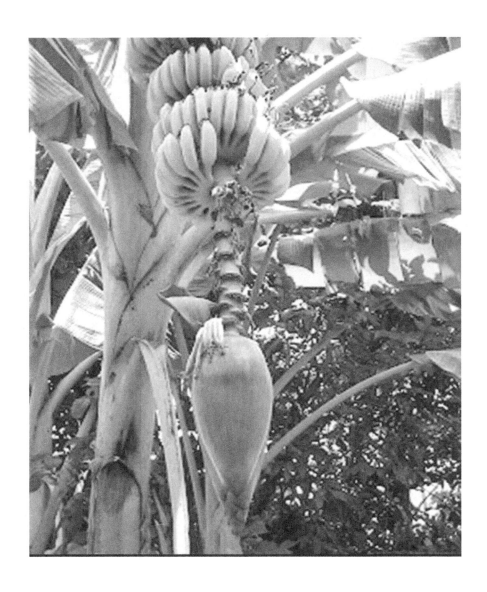

CHAPTER 2

RECOMMENDED DAILY FIBER

INTAKE

The recommended daily fiber intake varies based on factors such as age, gender, and overall health. The general guidelines provided by health organizations offer a framework for individuals to ensure they are meeting their nutritional needs. Fiber requirements are typically expressed in grams per day, and it's important to note that the recommendations might change as people age.

General Guidelines for Recommended Daily Fiber Intake:

The American Heart Association and the Institute of Medicine offer general guidelines for daily fiber intake:

- **Adult Men (18 years and older):** 38 grams per day

- **Adult Women (18 years and older):** 25 grams per day

These recommendations aim to support overall health, digestive function, and disease prevention. However, individual needs may vary based on factors like activity level, body weight, and specific health conditions.

Age and Gender-specific Recommendations:

1. **Children:**

   - Children aged 1-3 years: 19 grams per day

   - Children aged 4-8 years: 25 grams per day

   - Boys aged 9-13 years: 31 grams per day

   - Girls aged 9-13 years: 26 grams per day

   - Boys aged 14-18 years: 38 grams per day

   - Girls aged 14-18 years: 26 grams per day

2. **Adults:**

   - Men aged 19-50 years: 38 grams per day

   - Women aged 19-50 years: 25 grams per day

   - Men aged 51 years and older: 30 grams per day

   - Women aged 51 years and older: 21 grams per day

These recommendations serve as general guidelines, and individual needs may vary. Pregnant and breastfeeding women also have specific nutritional requirements, and it's advisable to consult with healthcare professionals for personalized guidance.

It's important to achieve the recommended fiber intake through a variety of food sources, including whole grains, fruits, vegetables, legumes, nuts, and seeds. Gradually increasing fiber intake and staying well-hydrated are essential to help prevent digestive discomfort associated with sudden dietary changes.

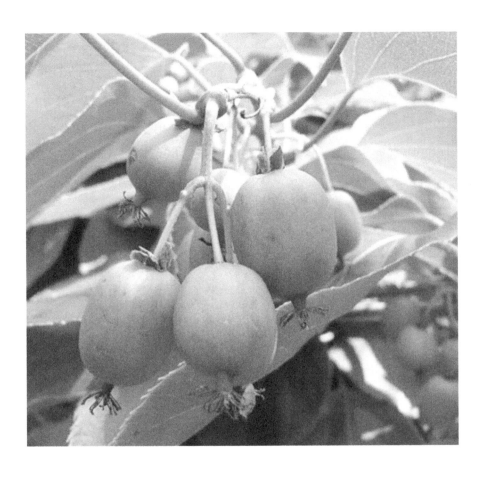

CHAPTER 3

HIGH-FIBER VEGETABLES

1. **Artichokes:**

    - Fiber: 5.4 grams

    - Calories: 47

    - Protein: 3.3 grams

    - Carbohydrates: 10.5 grams

    - Fat: 0.2 grams

    - Vitamins and minerals: Rich in vitamin C, vitamin K, folate, magnesium, and potassium.

2. **Broccoli:**

- Fiber: 2.6 grams

- Calories: 55

- Protein: 3.7 grams

- Carbohydrates: 11.2 grams

- Fat: 0.6 grams

- Vitamins and minerals: Excellent source of vitamin C, vitamin K, folate, and a good source of iron.

3. **Brussels Sprouts:**

- Fiber: 3.8 grams

- Calories: 43

- Protein: 3.4 grams

- Carbohydrates: 8.9 grams

- Fat: 0.3 grams

- Vitamins and minerals: High in vitamin K, vitamin C, vitamin A, and antioxidants.

4. **Carrots:**

- Fiber: 2.8 grams

- Calories: 41

- Protein: 0.9 grams

- Carbohydrates: 10 grams

- Fat: 0.2 grams

- Vitamins and minerals: Packed with beta-carotene, vitamin K, potassium, and vitamin B6.

5. **Lentils:**

- Fiber: 7.9 grams

- Calories: 116

- Protein: 9 grams

- Carbohydrates: 20 grams

- Fat: 0.4 grams

- Vitamins and minerals: Excellent source of iron, folate, manganese, and phosphorus.

6. **Peas:**

- Fiber: 5.5 grams

- Calories: 81

- Protein: 5.4 grams

- Carbohydrates: 14.5 grams

- Fat: 0.4 grams

- Vitamins and minerals: Good source of vitamin K, vitamin C, folate, and manganese.

7. **Spinach:**

- Fiber: 2.2 grams

- Calories: 23

- Protein: 2.9 grams

- Carbohydrates: 3.6 grams

- Fat: 0.4 grams

- Vitamins and minerals: High in iron, vitamin K, vitamin A, vitamin C, and folate.

8. **Sweet Potatoes:**

- Fiber: 3.0 grams

- Calories: 86

- Protein: 1.6 grams

- Carbohydrates: 20.1 grams

- Fat: 0.1 grams

- Vitamins and minerals: Rich in beta-carotene (vitamin A precursor), vitamin C, and potassium.

9. **Artichokes:**

- Fiber: 5.4 grams

- Calories: 47

- Protein: 3.3 grams

- Carbohydrates: 10.5 grams

- Fat: 0.2 grams

- Vitamins and minerals: Good source of antioxidants, vitamin C, vitamin K, and folate.

10. **Cauliflower:**

- Fiber: 2.0 grams

- Calories: 25

- Protein: 1.9 grams

- Carbohydrates: 5.3 grams

- Fat: 0.3 grams

- Vitamins and minerals: Contains vitamin C, vitamin K, folate, and is low in calories.

CHAPTER 4

HIGH-FIBER FRUITS

1. **Raspberries:**

   - Fiber: 6.5 grams

   - Calories: 52

   - Vitamin C: 26.2 mg

   - Antioxidants: Rich in anthocyanins and quercetin.

2. **Blackberries:**

   - Fiber: 5.3 grams

   - Calories: 43

   - Vitamin C: 21 mg

   - Antioxidants: Contains anthocyanins and ellagic acid.

3. **Avocado:**

- Fiber: 6.7 grams

- Calories: 160

- Healthy Fats: Rich in monounsaturated fats.

- Vitamins: High in vitamin K, vitamin E, and vitamin C.

4. **Pears:**

- Fiber: 3.1 grams

- Calories: 57

- Vitamin C: 3.1 mg

- Minerals: Contains potassium and copper.

5. **Apples:**

- Fiber: 2.4 grams

- Calories: 52

- Vitamin C: 0.5 mg

- Antioxidants: Contains flavonoids and polyphenols.

6. **Figs:**

- Fiber: 2.9 grams

- Calories: 74

- Minerals: Good source of calcium, potassium, and manganese.

7. **Guava:**

- Fiber: 5.4 grams

- Calories: 68

- Vitamin C: 228 mg

- Antioxidants: Rich in flavonoids and carotenoids.

8. **Bananas:**

- Fiber: 2.6 grams

- Calories: 89

- Minerals: Good source of potassium and vitamin B6.

9. **Prunes (Dried Plums):**

- Fiber: 7.1 grams

- Calories: 240

- Minerals: Rich in potassium, magnesium, and vitamin K.

10. **Kiwi:**

- Fiber: 3.0 grams

- Calories: 61

- Vitamin C: 92 mg

- Antioxidants: Contains vitamin E and polyphenols.

CHAPTER 5

WHOLE GRAINS

1. **Quinoa:**

    - Fiber: 2.8 grams

    - Calories: 120

    - Protein: 4.0 grams

    - Carbohydrates: 21.3 grams

    - Healthy Fats: 1.9 grams

    - Minerals: Contains iron, magnesium, and manganese.

2. **Oats:**

- Fiber: 10.6 grams

- Calories: 389

- Protein: 16.9 grams

- Carbohydrates: 66.3 grams

- Healthy Fats: 6.9 grams

- Minerals: Rich in manganese, phosphorus, and magnesium.

3. **Barley:**

- Fiber: 2.0 grams

- Calories: 123

- Protein: 2.3 grams

- Carbohydrates: 28.9 grams

- Healthy Fats: 0.4 grams

- Minerals: Contains copper, selenium, and phosphorus.

4. **Brown Rice:**

- Fiber: 1.6 grams

- Calories: 111

- Protein: 2.6 grams

- Carbohydrates: 23.5 grams

- Healthy Fats: 0.9 grams

- Minerals: Good source of magnesium and phosphorus.

5. **Buckwheat:**

- Fiber: 10.0 grams

- Calories: 343

- Protein: 13.3 grams

- Carbohydrates: 71.5 grams

- Healthy Fats: 3.4 grams

- Minerals: Rich in manganese, copper, and magnesium.

6. **Farro:**

- Fiber: 3.5 grams

- Calories: 337

- Protein: 14.6 grams

- Carbohydrates: 69.4 grams

- Healthy Fats: 1.9 grams

- Minerals: Contains iron, magnesium, and zinc.

7. **Amaranth:**

- Fiber: 6.7 grams

- Calories: 371

- Protein: 13.6 grams

- Carbohydrates: 66.5 grams

- Healthy Fats: 7.0 grams

- Minerals: Rich in iron, magnesium, and phosphorus.

8. **Whole Wheat (including whole wheat bread):**

- Fiber: 6.9 grams

- Calories: 247

- Protein: 13.2 grams

- Carbohydrates: 49.6 grams

- Healthy Fats: 2.1 grams

- Minerals: Good source of manganese, selenium, and phosphorus.

9. **Spelt:**

- Fiber: 7.6 grams

- Calories: 338

- Protein: 14.6 grams

- Carbohydrates: 70.2 grams

- Healthy Fats: 2.4 grams

- Minerals: Contains iron, magnesium, and phosphorus.

10. **Millet:**

- Fiber: 8.5 grams

- Calories: 378

- Protein: 11.0 grams

- Carbohydrates: 73.9 grams

- Healthy Fats: 4.0 grams

- Minerals: Rich in magnesium, phosphorus, and manganese.

CHAPTER 6

LEGUMES AND BEANS

1. **Lentils:**

    - Fiber: 7.9 grams

    - Calories: 116

    - Protein: 9.0 grams

    - Carbohydrates: 20.1 grams

    - Healthy Fats: 0.4 grams

    - Minerals: Excellent source of iron, folate, and manganese.

2. **Chickpeas (Garbanzo Beans):**

    - Fiber: 7.6 grams

    - Calories: 164

    - Protein: 8.9 grams

    - Carbohydrates: 27.4 grams

    - Healthy Fats: 2.6 grams

    - Minerals: Rich in iron, phosphorus, and zinc.

3. **Black Beans:**

- Fiber: 8.7 grams

- Calories: 132

- Protein: 8.9 grams

- Carbohydrates: 23.6 grams

- Healthy Fats: 0.5 grams

- Minerals: Good source of iron, magnesium, and phosphorus.

4. **Kidney Beans:**

- Fiber: 8.7 grams

- Calories: 127

- Protein: 8.7 grams

- Carbohydrates: 22.8 grams

- Healthy Fats: 0.5 grams

- Minerals: Contains iron, magnesium, and potassium.

5. **Split Peas:**

- Fiber: 8.3 grams

- Calories: 116

- Protein: 8.3 grams

- Carbohydrates: 20.4 grams

- Healthy Fats: 0.4 grams

- Minerals: Excellent source of iron, folate, and manganese.

6. **Pinto Beans:**

- Fiber: 9.0 grams

- Calories: 143

- Protein: 9.0 grams

- Carbohydrates: 26.2 grams

- Healthy Fats: 0.9 grams

- Minerals: Good source of iron, magnesium, and phosphorus.

7. **Black-eyed Peas:**

- Fiber: 6.7 grams

- Calories: 120

- Protein: 8.7 grams

- Carbohydrates: 23.0 grams

- Healthy Fats: 0.6 grams

- Minerals: Contains iron, magnesium, and potassium.

8. **Cannellini Beans:**

- Fiber: 6.4 grams

- Calories: 127

- Protein: 8.5 grams

- Carbohydrates: 23.1 grams

- Healthy Fats: 0.5 grams

- Minerals: Good source of iron, magnesium, and potassium.

9. **Adzuki Beans:**

- Fiber: 7.3 grams

- Calories: 128

- Protein: 7.5 grams

- Carbohydrates: 25.0 grams

- Healthy Fats: 0.5 grams

- Minerals: Rich in iron, potassium, and zinc.

10. **Chia Seeds:**

- Fiber: 34.4 grams

- Calories: 486

- Protein: 16.5 grams

- Carbohydrates: 42.1 grams

- Healthy Fats: 30.7 grams

- Minerals: Excellent source of omega-3 fatty acids, calcium, and manganese.

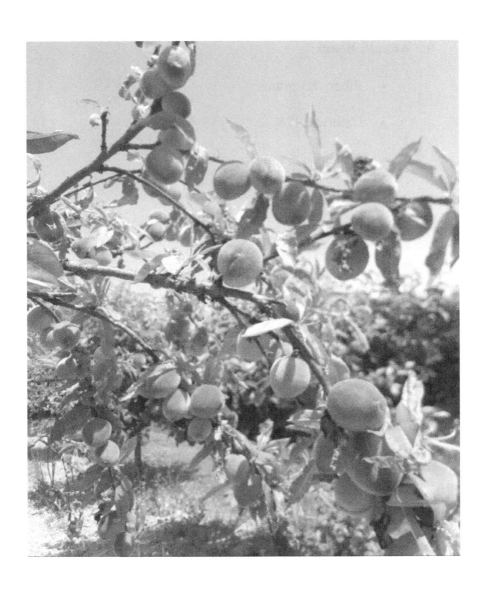

CHAPTER 7

NUTS AND SEEDS

1. **Flaxseeds:**

    - Fiber: 27.3 grams

    - Calories: 534

    - Protein: 18.3 grams

    - Carbohydrates: 28.9 grams

    - Healthy Fats: 42.2 grams

    - Minerals: Rich in omega-3 fatty acids, manganese, and magnesium.

2. **Sunflower Seeds:**

- Fiber: 8.6 grams

- Calories: 584

- Protein: 20.8 grams

- Carbohydrates: 23.7 grams

- Healthy Fats: 51.5 grams

- Minerals: Good source of vitamin E, copper, and selenium.

3. **Pumpkin Seeds (Pepitas):**

- Fiber: 5.0 grams

- Calories: 559

- Protein: 30.2 grams

- Carbohydrates: 10.7 grams

- Healthy Fats: 49.0 grams

- Minerals: Rich in magnesium, iron, and zinc.

4. **Almonds:**

- Fiber: 12.2 grams

- Calories: 576

- Protein: 21.2 grams

- Carbohydrates: 21.7 grams

- Healthy Fats: 49.4 grams

- Minerals: Excellent source of vitamin E, magnesium, and calcium.

5. **Walnuts:**

- Fiber: 6.7 grams

- Calories: 654

- Protein: 15.2 grams

- Carbohydrates: 13.7 grams

- Healthy Fats: 65.2 grams

- Minerals: Rich in omega-3 fatty acids, manganese, and copper.

6. **Pecans:**

- Fiber: 9.6 grams

- Calories: 691

- Protein: 9.2 grams

- Carbohydrates: 13.9 grams

- Healthy Fats: 71.2 grams

- Minerals: Good source of manganese, copper, and zinc.

7. **Brazil Nuts:**

- Fiber: 7.5 grams

- Calories: 656

- Protein: 14.3 grams

- Carbohydrates: 11.7 grams

- Healthy Fats: 66.4 grams

- Minerals: Rich in selenium, magnesium, and copper.

8. **Hazelnuts:**

- Fiber: 9.7 grams

- Calories: 628

- Protein: 15.0 grams

- Carbohydrates: 16.7 grams

- Healthy Fats: 60.8 grams

- Minerals: Good source of vitamin E, manganese, and copper.

9. **Cashews:**

- Fiber: 3.3 grams

- Calories: 553

- Protein: 18.2 grams

- Carbohydrates: 30.2 grams

- Healthy Fats: 43.9 grams

- Minerals: Contains iron, magnesium, and zinc.

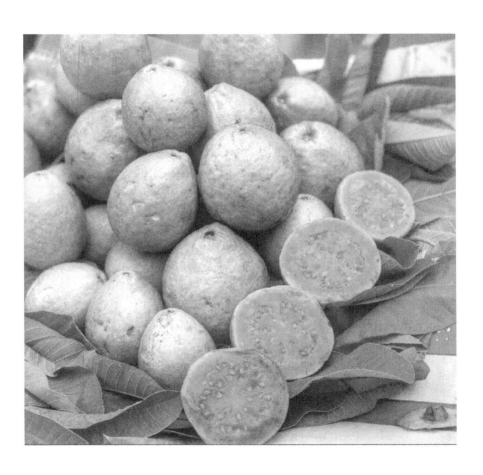

CHAPTER 8

FIBER-RICH SNACKS

1. **Popcorn:**

   - Fiber: 3.6 grams per 3 cups (popped)

   - Calories: 93

   - Protein: 3.1 grams

   - Carbohydrates: 18.7 grams

   - Healthy Fats: 1.2 grams

2. **Trail Mix with Nuts and Dried Fruits:**

   - Fiber: Varies (approximately 2-3 grams per 1/4 cup)

   - Calories: Varies

   - Protein: Varies

   - Carbohydrates: Varies

   - Healthy Fats: Varies

3. **Whole Grain Crackers with Hummus:**

- Fiber: Varies (approximately 2-3 grams per serving)

- Calories: Varies

- Protein: Varies

- Carbohydrates: Varies

- Healthy Fats: Varies

4. **Greek Yogurt with Berries:**

- Fiber: 2.6 grams per 1/2 cup (plain Greek yogurt)

- Calories: 59

- Protein: 10 grams

- Carbohydrates: 3.6 grams

- Healthy Fats: 0.4 grams

5. **Vegetable Sticks with Guacamole:**

- Fiber: Varies (approximately 3-4 grams per 1/2 cup guacamole)

- Calories: Varies

- Protein: Varies

- Carbohydrates: Varies

- Healthy Fats: Varies

6. **Roasted Chickpeas:**

- Fiber: 6.0 grams per 1/2 cup (roasted)

- Calories: 134

- Protein: 6.0 grams

- Carbohydrates: 19.8 grams

- Healthy Fats: 3.0 grams

7. **Apple Slices with Peanut Butter:**

    - Fiber: 4.0 grams per medium apple

    - Calories: 95

    - Protein: 2.0 grams

    - Carbohydrates: 20.0 grams

    - Healthy Fats: 2.0 grams (from 1 tablespoon of peanut butter)

8. **Dark Chocolate Covered Almonds:**

    - Fiber: 3.5 grams per 1/4 cup

    - Calories: 200

    - Protein: 5.0 grams

    - Carbohydrates: 17.0 grams

    - Healthy Fats: 14.0 grams

9. **Cottage Cheese with Pineapple:**

- Fiber: 1.0 gram per 1/2 cup (cottage cheese)

- Calories: 97

- Protein: 11 grams

- Carbohydrates: 7.0 grams

- Healthy Fats: 2.0 grams

10. **Edamame:**

- Fiber: 5.0 grams per 1 cup (cooked)

- Calories: 188

- Protein: 18.5 grams

- Carbohydrates: 13.0 grams

- Healthy Fats: 8.0 grams

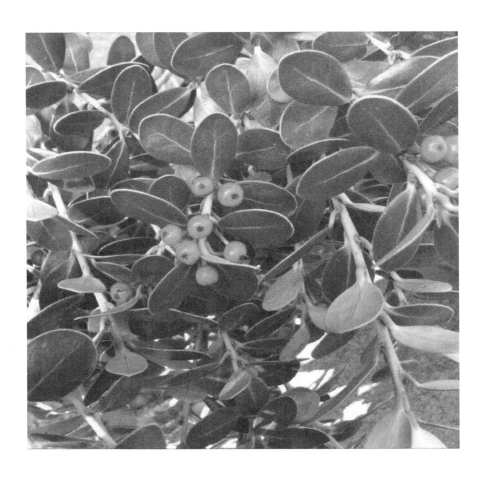

CONCLUSION

As we reach the closing chapter of this culinary exploration, I extend my heartfelt gratitude for joining me on this journey through the world of high-fiber foods. It has been my pleasure to guide you through the vibrant landscapes of nutrition, offering insights into the transformative power of dietary choices.

As we reflect on the benefits of incorporating high-fiber foods into our lives, I encourage you to consider the profound impact that each meal can have on your overall well-being. Picture a life where your energy soars, your digestion operates smoothly, and your mood is uplifted—all thanks to the choices you make on your plate. This is not an elusive dream but a tangible reality that awaits you.

The recipes presented in this book are more than just a collection of ingredients and instructions; they are a gateway to a healthier, more vibrant you. Each dish is a testament to the delicious possibilities that unfold when we prioritize the nutritional needs of our bodies. From quinoa salads to lentil soups, sweet potato tacos to chia seed puddings, these recipes are an invitation to savor the richness of life through the flavors of nourishing foods.

As you embark on your culinary adventure, I invite you to share your experiences and insights. Your feedback is a valuable ingredient in this ever-evolving recipe of knowledge. What recipes resonated with you? How did incorporating high-fiber foods into your diet impact your energy levels, digestion, and overall well-being? I am eager to hear your stories, your challenges, and your triumphs.

Remember, this journey is not a one-size-fits-all approach. It's about finding the flavors and combinations that resonate with your taste buds and nourish your unique body. Experiment with the recipes, add your personal touch, and make these dishes a reflection of your culinary preferences.

In closing, I want to express my sincere hope that this book has inspired you to view food not just as sustenance but as a source of vitality and joy. May each bite be a celebration of health, and may your journey toward a high-fiber lifestyle be filled with delicious discoveries.

Thank you for allowing me to be a part of your nutritional adventure. I look forward to hearing about your experiences, your triumphs in the kitchen, and the positive changes you witness on your journey to a healthier and more vibrant life.

BONUS CHAPTER 1

10 HIGH FIBER RECIPES

Quinoa Salad with Chickpeas and Vegetables

Cooking Time: 20 minutes

Servings: 4

Ingredients:

- 1 cup quinoa, rinsed

- 1 can chickpeas, drained and rinsed

- 1 cucumber, diced

- 1 bell pepper, diced

- 1 cup cherry tomatoes, halved

- 1/4 cup red onion, finely chopped

- 1/4 cup feta cheese, crumbled

- 2 tablespoons olive oil

- 1 lemon, juiced

- Salt and pepper to taste

Instructions:

1. Cook quinoa according to package instructions.

2. In a large bowl, combine cooked quinoa, chickpeas, cucumber, bell pepper, cherry tomatoes, red onion, and feta cheese.

3. In a small bowl, whisk together olive oil, lemon juice, salt, and pepper.

4. Drizzle the dressing over the salad and toss to combine.

5. Serve chilled.

Nutritional Information: Calories: 320 | Protein: 12g | Carbohydrates: 47g | Fiber: 10g | Fat: 12g

Lentil Soup

Cooking Time: 45 minutes

Servings: 6

Ingredients:

- 1 cup dried green lentils

- 1 onion, diced

- 2 carrots, diced

- 2 celery stalks, diced

- 3 cloves garlic, minced

- 1 can diced tomatoes

- 6 cups vegetable broth

- 1 teaspoon cumin

- 1 teaspoon coriander

- Salt and pepper to taste

- Fresh parsley for garnish

Instructions:

1. Rinse lentils under cold water.

2. In a large pot, sauté onion, carrots, and celery until softened.

3. Add garlic, lentils, diced tomatoes, vegetable broth, cumin, coriander, salt, and pepper.

4. Bring to a boil, then reduce heat and simmer for 30-35 minutes.

5. Garnish with fresh parsley before serving.

Nutritional Information: Calories: 240 | Protein: 14g | Carbohydrates: 40g | Fiber: 15g | Fat: 2g

Chickpea Stir-Fry

Cooking Time: 25 minutes

Servings: 4

Ingredients:

- 2 cans chickpeas, drained and rinsed

- 2 cups broccoli florets

- 1 bell pepper, sliced

- 1 carrot, julienned

- 2 tablespoons soy sauce

- 1 tablespoon olive oil

- 1 teaspoon ginger, minced

- 1 teaspoon garlic, minced

- 1 tablespoon sesame seeds for garnish

Instructions:

1. Heat olive oil in a pan, add ginger and garlic, sauté for 1 minute.

2. Add chickpeas, broccoli, bell pepper, and carrot. Cook until vegetables are tender.

3. Stir in soy sauce and cook for an additional 2-3 minutes.

4. Garnish with sesame seeds before serving.

Nutritional Information: Calories: 320 | Protein: 14g | Carbohydrates: 48g | Fiber: 12g | Fat: 9g

Sweet Potato and Black Bean Tacos

Cooking Time: 30 minutes

Servings: 4

Ingredients:

- 2 sweet potatoes, peeled and diced

- 1 can black beans, drained and rinsed

- 1 teaspoon cumin

- 1 teaspoon chili powder

- 1/2 teaspoon paprika

- 8 small whole wheat tortillas

- 1 cup salsa

- 1 avocado, sliced

- Fresh cilantro for garnish

Instructions:

1. Roast sweet potatoes in the oven at 400°F (200°C) for 20 minutes.

2. In a pan, heat black beans, cumin, chili powder, and paprika.

3. Warm tortillas and assemble tacos with roasted sweet potatoes, black beans, salsa, avocado, and cilantro.

Nutritional Information: Calories: 380 | Protein: 12g | Carbohydrates: 65g | Fiber: 14g | Fat: 10g

Spinach and Mushroom Quiche

Cooking Time: 50 minutes

Servings: 6

Ingredients:

- 1 whole wheat pie crust

- 4 cups fresh spinach

- 1 cup mushrooms, sliced

- 1 onion, diced

- 4 eggs

- 1 cup milk

- 1 cup feta cheese, crumbled

- Salt and pepper to taste

Instructions:

1. Preheat oven to 375°F (190°C).

2. Sauté mushrooms and onions until softened.

3. In a bowl, whisk together eggs, milk, salt, and pepper.

4. Layer spinach, sautéed mushrooms, and feta cheese in the pie crust.

5. Pour the egg mixture over the ingredients.

6. Bake for 35-40 minutes or until the center is set.

Nutritional Information: Calories: 280 | Protein: 12g | Carbohydrates: 20g | Fiber: 4g | Fat: 16g

Berry and Yogurt Parfait

Cooking Time: 10 minutes (assembly)
Servings: 2

Ingredients:

- 1 cup Greek yogurt

- 1 cup mixed berries (strawberries, blueberries, raspberries)

- 1/2 cup granola

- 2 tablespoons honey

Instructions:

1. In glasses or bowls, layer Greek yogurt, mixed berries, and granola.

2. Drizzle honey over the top.

3. Repeat the layers and finish with a drizzle of honey.

Nutritional Information: Calories: 280 | Protein: 18g | Carbohydrates: 48g | Fiber: 6g | Fat: 6g

Hummus and Veggie Wrap

Cooking Time: 10 minutes

Servings: 2

Ingredients:

- 4 whole wheat tortillas

- 1 cup hummus

- 1 cucumber, thinly sliced

- 1 bell pepper, thinly sliced

- 1 carrot, julienned

- Handful of spinach leaves

Instructions:

1. Spread hummus on each tortilla.

2. Layer with cucumber, bell pepper, carrot, and spinach.

3. Roll the tortillas tightly and cut in half.

Nutritional Information: Calories: 320 | Protein: 12g | Carbohydrates: 50g | Fiber: 10g | Fat: 10g

Brown Rice and Vegetable Stir-Fry

Cooking Time: 25 minutes

Servings: 4

Ingredients:

- 2 cups cooked brown rice

- 1 cup broccoli florets

- 1 bell pepper, sliced

- 1 carrot, julienned

- 1 zucchini, sliced

- 2 tablespoons low-sodium soy sauce

- 1 tablespoon sesame oil

- 1 teaspoon ginger, minced

- 1 teaspoon garlic, minced

- Sesame seeds for garnish

Instructions:

1. In a wok or large pan, heat sesame oil and sauté ginger and garlic.

2. Add vegetables and stir-fry until tender.

3. Stir in cooked brown rice and soy sauce.

4. Garnish with sesame seeds before serving.

Nutritional Information: Calories: 280 | Protein: 8g | Carbohydrates: 50g | Fiber: 8g | Fat: 6g

Apple and Almond Butter Sandwich

Preparation Time: 5 minutes

Servings: 1

Ingredients:

- 2 slices whole grain bread

- 1 medium apple, thinly sliced

- 2 tablespoons almond butter

- Cinnamon for sprinkling

Instructions:

1. Spread almond butter on one side of each bread slice.

2. Arrange apple slices on one bread slice and sprinkle with cinnamon.

3. Place the other bread slice on top, almond butter side down.

Nutritional Information: Calories: 320 | Protein: 8g | Carbohydrates: 50g | Fiber: 8g | Fat: 12g

Quinoa and Black Bean Stuffed Bell Peppers

Cooking Time: 40 minutes

Servings: 4

Ingredients:

- 4 bell peppers, halved and seeds removed

- 1 cup quinoa, cooked

- 1 can black beans, drained and rinsed

- 1 cup corn kernels

- 1 cup diced tomatoes

- 1 teaspoon cumin

- 1 teaspoon chili powder

- Salt and pepper to taste

- 1 cup shredded cheddar cheese

- Fresh cilantro for garnish

Instructions:

1. Preheat oven to 375°F (190°C).

2. In a bowl, mix cooked quinoa, black beans, corn, diced tomatoes, cumin, chili powder, salt, and pepper.

3. Stuff each bell pepper half with the quinoa mixture.

4. Top with shredded cheddar cheese.

5. Bake for 25-30 minutes or until peppers are tender.

6. Garnish with fresh cilantro before serving.

Nutritional Information: Calories: 340 | Protein: 15g | Carbohydrates: 55g | Fiber: 12g | Fat: 8g

IF YOU WANT MORE RECIPES, YOU CAN CHECK OUT

OTHER BOOKS BY THE AUTHOR

GLUTEN-FREE COOKBOOK FOR VEGAN

GLUTEN-FREE INSTANT POT COOKBOOK

TYPE 2 DIABETES COOKBOOK FOR SENI0RS

MEDITERRANEAN SLOW COOKER COOKBOOK FOR

WOMEN

LOW SODIUM COOKBOOK FOR BEGINNERS

TO GET ACCESS TO MORE BOOKS BY THE AUTHOR

SCAN THE QR CODE

BONUS CHAPTER 2

21 DAY MEAL PLAN

Day	Breakfast	Lunch	Dinner	Snack
1	Greek Yogurt Parfait	Quinoa Salad with Chickpeas	Grilled Chicken with Roasted Veggies	Apple Slices with Peanut Butter
2	Oatmeal with Berries	Lentil Soup	Baked Salmon with Quinoa	Carrot Sticks with Hummus
3	Scrambled Eggs with Spinach	Hummus and Veggie Wrap	Sweet Potato and Black Bean Tacos	Mixed Nuts
4	Whole Grain Toast with Avocado	Brown Rice and Vegetable Stir-Fry	Spinach and Mushroom Quiche	Greek Yogurt with Berries

5	Chia Seed Pudding	Chickpea Stir-Fry	Stuffed Bell Peppers	Trail Mix
6	Apple and Almond Butter Sandwich	Black Bean Salad	Quinoa and Black Bean Stew	Cottage Cheese with Pineapple
7	Banana Walnut Muffins	Vegetable and Lentil Curry	Grilled Turkey Burgers	Dark Chocolate Covered Almonds
8	Berry Smoothie Bowl	Baked Sweet Potato Fries	Shrimp and Broccoli Stir-Fry	Edamame
9	Whole Wheat Pancakes with Berries	Caprese Salad with Whole Wheat Bread	Turkey and Vegetable Skewers	Greek Yogurt Parfait
10	Avocado and Tomato Toast	Quinoa and Black Bean Burrito Bowl	Baked Chicken with Brown Rice	Roasted Chickpeas

11	Overnight Oats with Almond Butter	Lentil and Vegetable Stir-Fry	Grilled Portobello Mushrooms	Trail Mix
12	Spinach and Feta Omelette	Black Bean and Corn Quesadillas	Teriyaki Salmon with Quinoa	Carrot Sticks with Hummus
13	Yogurt and Fruit Smoothie	Hummus and Avocado Wrap	Chickpea and Vegetable Curry	Mixed Nuts
14	Quinoa Breakfast Bowl	Roasted Vegetable Salad	Baked Zucchini Boats	Dark Chocolate Covered Almonds
15	Peanut Butter Banana Toast	Lentil and Spinach Stuffed Peppers	Grilled Chicken Caesar Salad	Greek Yogurt with Berries
16	Chia Seed Pudding	Sweet Potato and Black Bean Salad	Quinoa and Veggie Stir-Fry	Cottage Cheese with Pineapple

17	Whole Grain Waffles with Strawberries	Chickpea and Spinach Salad	Baked Cod with Brown Rice	Apple Slices with Peanut Butter
18	Breakfast Burrito	Lentil Soup	Turkey and Quinoa Stuffed Peppers	Edamame
19	Greek Yogurt Parfait	Quinoa Salad with Chickpeas	Grilled Vegetable Skewers	Trail Mix
20	Oatmeal with Almond Butter	Brown Rice and Black Bean Bowl	Baked Chicken with Quinoa	Mixed Nuts
21	Scrambled Eggs with Avocado	Hummus and Veggie Wrap	Grilled Salmon with Roasted Veggies	Dark Chocolate Covered Almonds